MOTIVATIONAL STRENGTH

LEARN TO STRENGTHEN YOUR MOTIVATIONAL HABITS TO CONTINUE REACHING YOUR HEALTH AND FITNESS GOALS

By Coach Blaire Camarda, CPT, CSCS

Founder of

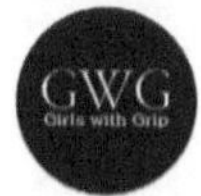

First paperback edition July 2020

Imprint: Independently published

Book design and cover design by Ana Kreker

ISBN 9798665292656

THE STUFF IN THIS BOOK

WHAT IS
GIRLS WITH
GRIP

Girls with Grip is a community of like-minded women looking to strengthen all areas of their lives. This is a place for women who want to learn more about strength training, strength sports, and how to be their own version of an ultimate badass! The physical strength of a woman used to be very taboo, but those days are gone, and we want to celebrate this time.

In this community, we delve into different aspects of strength to add to your arsenal and ways to gain strength, so you get the most out of a fitness or strength workout program. In this series, we discuss topics such as, how to create motivation from within, how confidence increases strength, and how emotional tenacity surfaces in workouts.

This is a time to be celebrated and we Girls with Grip are so happy you have decided to join us. To interact with us daily, follow us on Instagram (@girlswithgrip). If you are positive and looking to contribute to creating mutual badassery within this community of women, we hope you will join us!

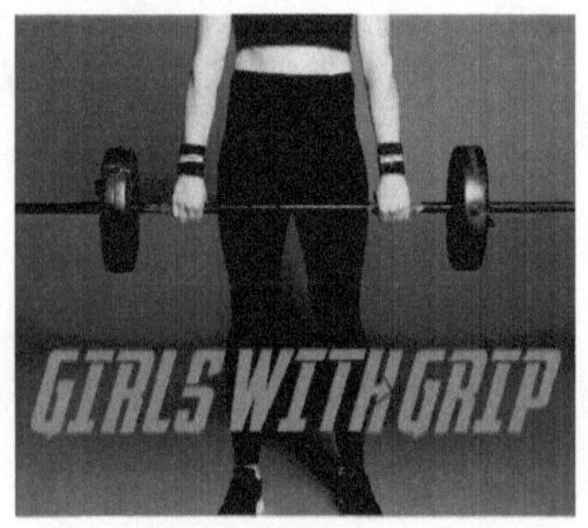

How to contact Girls with Grip:

IG: @girlswithgrip

Email: girlswithgrip@outlook.com

LOVE, COACH BLAIRE

Dear Reader,

Let's start with a little about me so you aren't talking to a stranger. My name is Blaire Camarda and I live with fibromyalgia and chronic pelvic issues.

Fibromyalgia. The word that changed every aspect of my life. Full-body physical pain, 24/7. It is exhausting. Always feeling on the verge of the flu, but it does not come. It is frustrating. Learning there is no cure. It is defeating. I experience varying levels of chronic pain throughout my body, extreme fatigue, migraines, bloating, pelvic pain, irregular body temperature, weight gain and more—but you get the idea. Growing up playing sports through college and then continuing my professional career in health, fitness and athletic development all I have ever known is being active to some degree and did not really start to struggle with or my get my diagnosis until my early thirties. I didn't understand why I always felt sick when I was active and ate healthy food. It will suck the motivation and life right out of you!

I have overcome injuries and surgeries courtesy of contact sports, but this was different. I had to develop a new understanding of how to stay motivated; how to work with (not against) my physical limitations and adversities. These are all things I never thought I would experience. After years of being poked, prodded, examined, and told there was nothing each doctor could do for me, I had two choices. I could continue the vicious cycle of insanity, inconclusive test results and disappointment OR I could become my own best advocate, let go of what I cannot control, and get the most out of my life by focusing on the things I can control. I chose option two.

This meant, I had to get comfortable learning how to work in harmony with my circumstances <u>to provide myself the opportunity to continue moving forward. In turn, it has affected my emotional, mental, and spiritual strength in a great way.</u>

P.S. This book is not about fibromyalgia ☻

To strengthen my motivation, I aim to keep a schedule, stay organized and prepared the best I can, and remind myself that even if I don't feel great due to my medical "stuff" that staying active is still helping me, in the long run, to increase my tolerance, reduce stress and manage my symptoms. This process is always an uphill battle and, honestly, difficult to maintain. But I focus on the steps laid out in this book to support my goals and give myself a chance to get the most of my strength program.

My circumstances may be different from yours, but we all have them. How we CHOOSE to handle our circumstances, directly effects our outcomes. We have all heard the saying "our lives are 10% what happens to us and 90% how we react to it". If you haven't yet gotten the memo…consider the memo delivered. BECAUSE IT'S TRUE.

This is your opportunity to regain and strengthen your sense of self, take more control over your life, and reach potential in the ways you seek. It IS possible!

I invite you to dig deep and put in the effort you deserve to jump start your progress and change your life. I hope this book provides a platform to tap into your inner strength, keep your personal power and create your own motivation. It's time to get motivated and crush goals!

Love, Coach Blaire

ACKNOWLEDGMENT

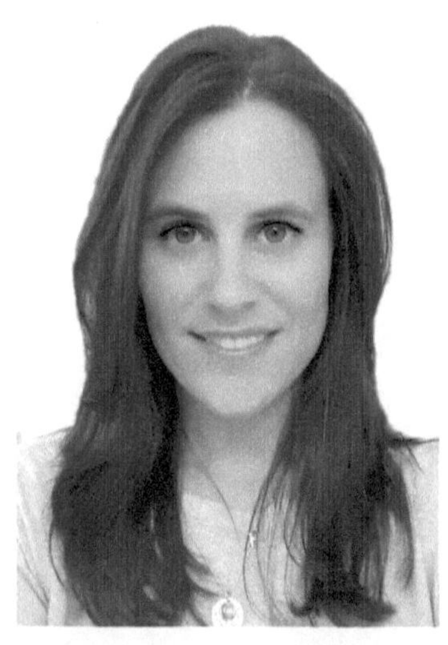

Before we start this journey, I want to thank all my clients who have felt comfortable enough to share, been willing to tap into their own potential and strengthen their own motivational habits by connecting to their experiences and facing their obstacles by committing to overcome them. Only when you committed, did you create action to breed your personal motivation. Thank you for going for it! You are the true inspiration for this book.

I would also like to thank those that helped make this book come to life. Thanks to my family (Mom, Dad, Al, and Court), Tanya, Tammy, and Jay for the time spent providing feedback and support during this process. To Anastasia for making this thing REAL! I've learned much from you and can't wait for what's next. To Coach Glabb, for the guidance, support, and belief in me and my ability to tackle this project—I couldn't have done it without your suggestions and tools. This is where it all started and I couldn't have done it without any of you.

FIRST AND FOREMOST

Preface

For a moment, let's talk stressors. This word encompasses mental, physical, emotional or spiritual stressors and tends to create unforeseen obstacles or makes adhering to a health and fitness program a bit more involved. It is not always as simple as getting your workout in. The workout is static, it does not have feelings and it did not choose you; you must choose it. That choice requires action and when we take that action it becomes a bit easier to see our workouts through.

We all have struggles PLUS the ability to commit to strengthening our motivational habits. Do not ever forget you have this ability. It is the foundation of your personal power and the creation of your motivation. This relationship between our stressors and how we choose to handle them, makes all the difference in the world.

What you take away from this experience is up to you. The way to get the most out of this book is to approach it with an open mind and a willingness to assess yourself.

Self-awareness is the key to strengthening your motivational habits. Acknowledge where you are, why you are there, and how high your health and wellness rank on your personal list of priorities.

IT IS A DECISION!

First and foremost, get yourself in a mindset to accept new information and be willing to make some changes so you can create your motivation in ways you never have before.

The **willingness** is the secret sauce when it comes to making lasting changes.

DON'T DOWNGRADE YOUR DREAM JUST TO FIT YOUR REALITY.

UPGRADE YOUR CONVICTION TO MATCH YOUR DESTINY.

If improving your health, wellness and every version of your strength is a priority then you are primed and ready to see some seriously cool improvements when it comes to being a badass!

At this moment if you have doubts, concerns or questions, write them down! As you go through this book, check the items off your lists and make notes as they are addressed. Use the guide below to help organize your thoughts, concerns, fears, and questions. You don't need to fill in every line and/or you can fill in more. Use the guide to fit your needs. Be sure to identify WHY you have the concerns and fears you are experiencing. There is not a wrong answer and the identification of these reasons is a game-changer, so don't skip this section. At the end, if there are any areas not addressed or you would like additional information, please reach out to us directly at girlswithgrip@outlook.com.

Let's quickly breakdown how to tackle each of these areas.

Your thoughts and opinions are your initial thoughts on how you think your experience will be or how you hope your motivation will be influenced by this book. Write them in the following table.

My **thoughts/opinions** around creating my own motivation are:

Questions are vital to acknowledge. Without the clarity and identification of what you are wondering about, you will not be able to check items off, at the end, to know if your questions have been answered. Write them in the following table.

My **questions** around creating my own motivation are:
☐ 1.
☐ 2.
☐ 3.
☐ 4.

Addressing fears and concerns is two-fold. First, identify the actual fear concisely. Then, acknowledge WHY you have this fear. Simple, right? If you feel overwhelmed, not to worry! There is no wrong fear and no wrong reason why — everything you write is correct. This can be uncomfortable and even feel a bit vulnerable, but you are here for a reason. Get everything you can out of this book so you can crush it! Own what you are experiencing so it can be addressed, and you can continue moving forward. Fill in as few or as many (or more!) as you like. Write your concise fears and concerns in the following table.

My **concerns/fears** around creating my own motivation are:
☐ 1.
☐ 2.
☐ 3.
☐ 4.

Now, match each fear or concern with a reason. For example: if my fear was "I will fail and not be able to create my motivation", (now, I need to ask myself why?) and I would identify the reason as, "I don't believe I can meet my goals". Allow yourself to be uncomfortable — that's how you know you are allowing yourself the opportunity to change and to improve. Write your reasons in the following table.

I have these **concerns/fears** because:
☐ 1.
☐ 2.
☐ 3.
☐ 4.

Take a deep breath and relax, the tough part is over.

Now, we are ready to get into the meat and potatoes (YUM!) about how to strengthen your own motivational habits!

MAKE DECISIONS

We are getting right to it with a truth bomb! YOU WILL NOT ALWAYS FEEL MOTIVATED! There it is — just like pulling off a band-aid and now we can get to work.

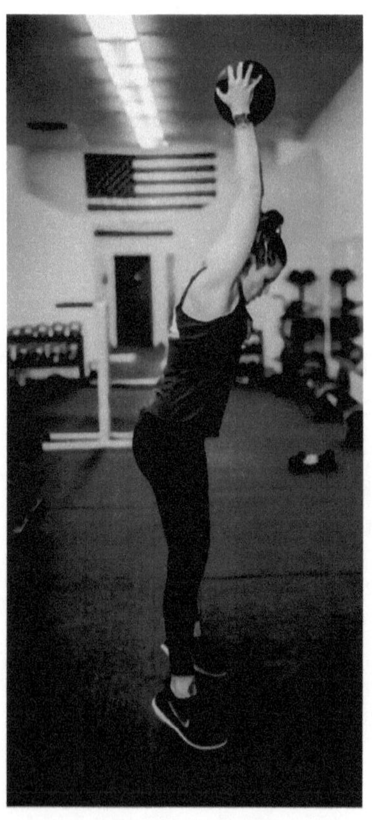

When we set goals, we have an idea (or hope...) of smoothness along the way or at the start of our health and fitness journey. Sometimes we don't factor in our responses to obstacles and adversities. We are constantly faced with forks in the road and if we don't decide which direction to go our goals become roadkill.

What do your obstacles look like?

Maybe outside factors such as work obligations or last-minute duties with a spouse or for your children pop up unexpectedly.

Maybe your eating was off today, so you figure you will get back on track tomorrow.

Maybe you have a chronic illness or chronic pain that makes any sort of a plan difficult to adhere too and you are just plain irritated with everything. Don't worry, it happens!

Whatever your obstacles look like, identify and write them in the following table.

My *obstacles*:
1.
2.
3.
4.

No matter what the obstacle, there is a way to find your motivation and overcome it. But first, you must decide to act!

When we have authentic intention, have set clear goals and laid out a progressive plan, we must be prepared to act. But how? Keep it simple. Eat the vegetables instead of the fries or maybe you only have 65% to give to your workout, today — be sure to give 100% of that 65%. We must CHOOSE to be about it, not just speak about it.

No one feels completely motivated all the time and you are not alone (if anyone says otherwise, they are lying to your face). Remember that a little planning, a few deep breaths and a commitment to decision goes a very long way!

DECIDE TO TAKE ACTION WHEN YOU ARE NOT FEELING INNATELY MOTIVATED.

TAKE ACTION

Let's Review

Motivation does not exist without a little self-discipline, progressive planning, goal setting, and a WILLINGNESS TO TAKE ACTION.

Willingness and decision to take one positive action step, in times when motivation feels low, will keep you on track. This prevents "restarting" and creates an environment of consistency that lays the foundation for you to reach your health and fitness goals. Your ultimate objective is to learn how to keep your motivation in homeostasis when it might otherwise be low.

Strengthening motivational habits requires action and planning!

ACTION 1: Decide to PRIORITIZE

ACTION 2: Decide to find a COACH

ACTION 3: Decide to TRACK

ACTION 4: Decide to FOSTER

ACTION 5: Decide to FORGET

ACTION 1: Decide to PRIORITIZE

Decide your workouts and meal planning are the same priority level as an appointment you would not cancel (doctor, dentist, etc.). These appointments are crucial to your progress — don't cancel them! See the following two examples for monthly and weekly calendar versions.

MONTH						
Sunday	**Monday**	**Tuesday**	**Wednesday**	**Thursday**	**Friday**	**Saturday**
☐	☐	☐	☐	☐	☐	☐
☐	☐	☐	☐	☐	☐	☐
☐	☐	☐	☐	☐	☐	☐
☐	☐	☐	☐	☐	☐	☐
☐	☐	☐	☐	☐	☐	☐

For the weekly version, you can include all seven days of the week or your five busiest days to keep it simple, manageable, and more focused at the start. On these calendars, at least fill in your workout times and meal prep times.

Monday Date:		Tuesday Date:		Wednesday Date:		Thursday Date:		Friday Date	
8		8		8		8		8	
A		A		A		A		A	
9		9		9		9		9	
A		A		A		A		A	
10		10		10		10		10	
A		A		A		A		A	
11		11		11		11		11	
A		A		A		A		A	
12		12		12		12		12	
P		P		P		P		P	
1		1		1		1		1	
P		P		P		P		P	
2		2		2		2		2	
P		P		P		P		P	
3		3		3		3		3	
P		P		P		P		P	
4		4		4		4		4	
P		P		P		P		P	
5		5		5		5		5	
P		P		P		P		P	
6		6		6		6		6	
P		P		P		P		P	
	Evening		Evening		Evening		Evening		Evening

ACTION 2: Decide to find a COACH

Work with a coach you trust and who has your best interest at the forefront. Even though the process and journey are yours, we get further with a support system. If you start working with a coach and you realize at any point it is not a good fit for you, be willing to move on and find the right person to help support your progress. Remember, any coach you choose cannot make these changes for you. He/she should be a support beam in your foundation during this process—adding to your experience. In the end, it is within your power!

Some questions to ask yourself when choosing a coach:

1. Does this person have my best interest at the forefront?

2. Is this person taking the time to fully understand my obstacles and fears?

3. Do I believe we will work well together?

4. Am I comfortable being uncomfortable and am I willing to commit to my program?

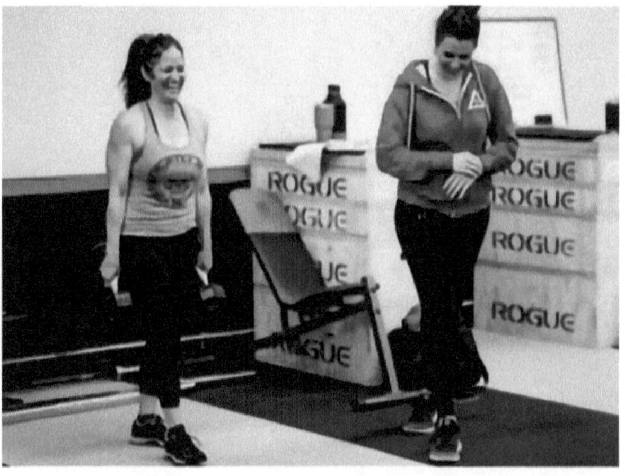

ACTION 3: Decide to TRACK

Use a tracking system. By trial and error, find the system that works best for you; whether it be old school paper and pen, an online tracking system or an accountability coach you trust. Be willing to try and try again! It is important to track your workouts and reflect on the results periodically so you and your coach can identify where, if any, course corrections are needed. This is not a time of judgment or comparison. This is a time to allow you the opportunity to minimize setbacks and maximize progress! A tool such as this should be supplied by your coach. If it's not, use this one! See the items below with a super simple way to track them.

Exercise and Fitness: 3 ways you will improve your exercise and fitness

1) ____

2) ____

3) ____

Date to review: ____

Action steps accomplished? (yes/no, explain)

____

____

____

Course corrections to add with new date to evaluate:

____

____

____

Follow the above breakdown for the following categories:

- Nutrition and hydration

- Obstacle identification

- Ways to overcome obstacles

Create this system to fit your needs and goals. It is yours to craft!

ACTION 4: Decide to FOSTER

Foster your mental, emotional and spiritual strength. Find a great book, podcast, YouTube channel or local seminar to attend for additional motivational guidance. There are many great choices!

Here is a short list of personal development books, I love, to help get you started (most are audio books as well):

1. Mind Gym: An Athlete's Guide to Inner Excellence, Gary Mack

2. UnFu*K Yourself: Get Out of Your Head and Into Your Life, Gary John Bishop

3. 10% Happier, Dan Harris

4. The 7 Habits of Highly Effective People, Stephen Covey

5. You Are a Badass, Jen Sincero

MOTIVATION DRILL DOWN

Five actions steps to breed your motivation

ACTION 1: PRIORITIZE

ACTION 2: COACH

ACTION 3: TRACK

ACTION 4: FOSTER

ACTION 5: FORGET

HELPFUL HINTS:

1. Work on one action step at a time so you gradually build a foundation until all five steps are working together and synchronized.

2. Be willing to make mistakes. It is the ONLY way to find the plan of attack that works best for you (AKA "trial and error"). If there was one cookie-cutter process that worked across the board, we would all be using it.

3. Terminate the "start over" mentality. Simply work to "course correct" as obstacles arise, or you stumble upon something that isn't working. Get back on track, assess at your milestones, and don't throw all your progress out the window by starting over. Keep going.

ACTION 5: Decide to FORGET

Be willing to forget everything you know about what you are "supposed to do". We see so many images and motivational quotes on social media (not all real BTW) that we often don't realize we have pre-formulated an expectation of what we should look like, how long it should take to get there, and how easy the process will be. You are your own blank canvas; you can create your piece of art any way you choose...with zero comparison to anyone else.

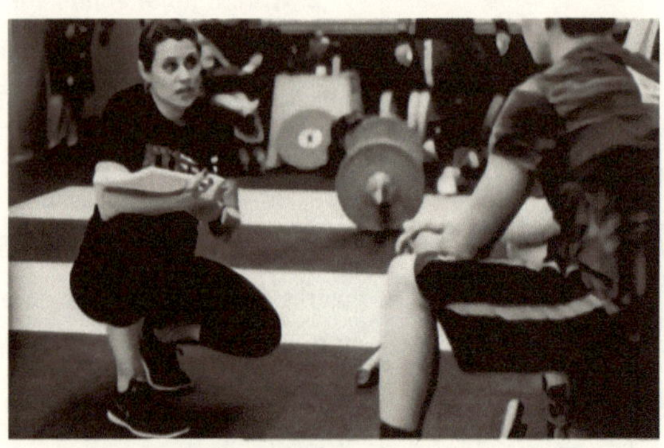

At the end of the day, (1) keep your motivation a priority, and (2) decide to not quit. With these two pieces of the equation locked in, the rest (workout, meal planning, confidence, self-awareness, etc.) will fall into place over time. It's not always sexy, but it is THE WAY to strengthen motivational habits and continue crushing your goals!

RECAP TIME

- How we CHOOSE to handle our circumstances, directly effects our outcomes. The saying "our lives are 10% what happens to us and 90% how we react to it" IS TRUE.

- Willingness to commit is the secret sauce when it comes to making lasting changes.

- YOU WILL NOT ALWAYS FEEL MOTIVATED! No one feels completely motivated all the time. Remember that a little planning, a few deep breaths and a commitment to decision breeds A LOT of motivation!

- Strengthening motivational habits requires action and planning!

ACTION 1: Decide to PRIORITIZE

ACTION 2: Decide to find a COACH

ACTION 3: Decide to TRACK

ACTION 4: Decide to FOSTER

ACTION 5: Decide to FORGET

- It's not always sexy, but THE WAY to create motivation and crush your goals is the decision to act when motivation feels low.

FINAL THOUGHTS

Now is the time to go back and revisit the doubts, concerns, and questions you recorded before we began. Review them. Have they been addressed? If so, this is the time to take one action step. Remember to pick one at a time and build up until you are actively working with all five action steps regularly. Which action step do you choose to start with?

My first action step: _______________________________________

If your fears, concerns, or questions were not answered—let me know! Everyone has a different experience and different needs to be filled with strengthening motivational habits. It is up to you (and me, if you let me know ☺) to discover what you need to customize these action steps, so you continue your forward progress with a deeper understanding of your motivational strength.

To close, thank you for reading this book. I hope you have gained a few nuggets to take away and apply when your motivational tank is not full. I want to hear how this information has helped you or if you have additional questions about strengthening your motivation. Please feel free to contact me directly at girlswithgrip@outlook.com. I want to know how your journey is going and what works for you. You will likely provide a nugget that can help someone else that we can include in the future with the 2nd edition ☺. Thank you for strengthening your badassery and elevating your motivational strength! Merry Motivation and Happy Goal Crushing!

Now is the time to take action. Don't wait. I look forward to hearing your success stories and answering your questions!

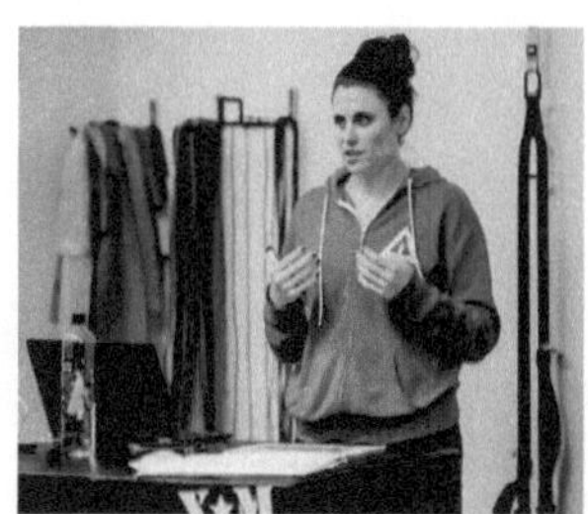

How to contact Girls with Grip:

IG: @girlswithgrip

Email: girlswithgrip@outlook.com

9 798665 292656